ELECTRICIAN'S PRAYER MANUAL SQUARED

Mountain = Djou

EnQi Osiris Kheper
Sang Real

Amazon

CONTENTS

INTRODUCTION

Pray or be Prey... Please we need God now and we need unity, black, white, tall, short, fat, skinny...

WELCOME

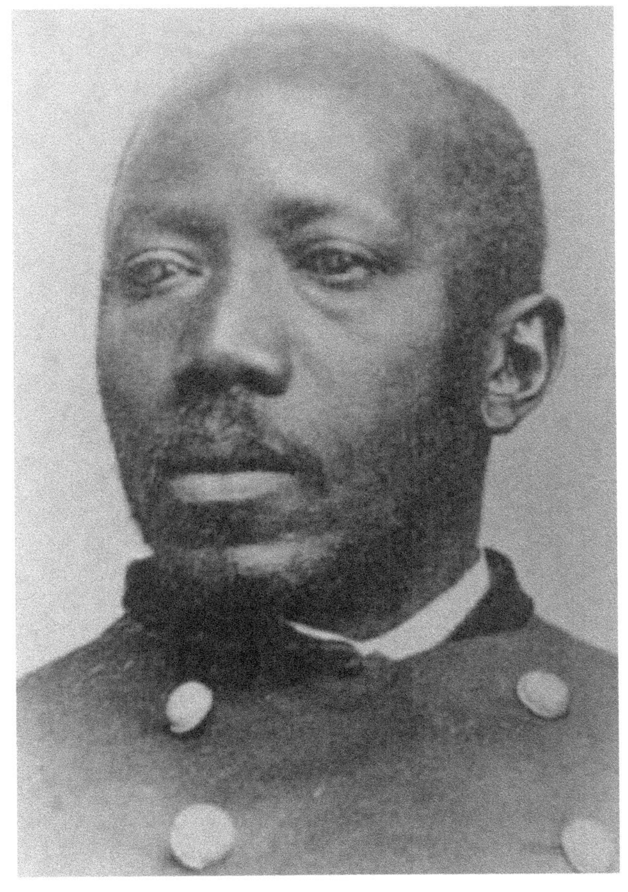

Martin Delany the first American to be fluent in Mdu Ntr, he was a medical doctor, politician, author, publisher, novelist, explorer, and army officer.

Psalms 68:31

Princes shall come out of Egypt; Ethiopia shall soon stretch out her hands unto God.

This verse from the Bible is often hidden, its very telling of the hidden communication encoded in the Bible. The same egyptologist have hidden Reeds & Feathers. Reeds and Feathers are the keys to Kemet, they have the same type of sounds, but Reeds refer to Men, Feathers refer to Gods. Reeds and Feathers have been slickly converted into the Yod, the trick is 800 glyphs can not be surmised by 22, 26 or 27... Those numbers have other meanings themselves... Common people will never know these things!

We have to take this serious...

Watch how one papyri puts all the con men, Satanists and misguided souls bed. The talking that 12,500 year old pyramid stuff... All to deny the Bros their legacy! The Diary of Merer (Khufu peeps), proof the Great Pyramid is Somolon temple of the Bible, the spot were Moses received the Law... This papyri proves the new agers are satanists! All the pyramid is 12,000 years old people like Billy, trying to slick 'discredit the Bible'... Busted!!! Well maybe it doesn't prove all that you Lmao... It at least proves Khufu did his thing! You would have to go to L'Goat book to get the reasons I have on Solomon's Temple, besides common sense. How are they writing a master piece of wisdom, in Egypt, that wouldn't include the Pyramids. They were more magical then, we have ruins now... Remember the Arabs & Muslims that ate the mummies, blew a hole in the pyramid in 820 ad, stole all the papyri and gold, creating the wealth they now pretend comes from oil! They have laundered the wealth of the Kemetyu (Kemetiyu) families, now struggling around the world to make ends meet. Think the "Age of Oil" began in the 1800s, Oil money is relatively new money!!! I live for the Day Black Billions launch the Restore the Pyramids Project! We should have never been on a return to Africa program, it should've always been return to Kemet & Nubia! Goofballs have been pimping Kemet for years, they could've been buying the land.

[First day] the director of 6 Idjer[u] casts of for Heliopolis in a transport boat-iuat to bring us food from Heliopolis while the Elite (stp-s3) is in Tura.
Day 2: Inspector Merer spends the day with his phyle hauling stones in Tura North; spends the night at Tura North.
Day 3: Inspector Merer casts off from Tura North, sails towards Akhet-Khufu loaded with stone.
[Day 4 ...] the director of 6 [Idjer]u [comes back] from

Heliopolis with 40 sacks-khar and a large measure-heqat of bread-beset while the Elite hauls stones in Tura North.

Day 5: Inspector Merer spends the day with his phyle loading stones onto the boats-hau of the Elite in Tura North, spends the night at Tura.

Day 6: Inspector Merer sets sail with a boat of the naval section (gs-dpt) of Ta-ur, going downriver towards Akhet-Khufu. Spends the night at Ro-She Khufu.

Day 7: sets sail in the morning towards Akhet-Khufu, sails towing towards Tura North, spends the night at […]

Day 8: sets sail from Ro-She Khufu, sails towards Tura North. Inspector Merer spends the day [with a boat?] of Ta-ur? […].

Day 9: sets sail from […] of Khufu […].

Day 10: […]

[Day 13 …] She-[Khufu] […] spends the night at Tur]a South.

[Day 14: … hauling] stones [… spends the night in] Tura South.

[Day 15:] Inspector Merer [spends the day] with his [phyle] hauling stones [in Tura] South, spends the night in Tura South.

[Day 16: Inspector Merer spends the day with] his phyle loading the boat-imu (?) with stone [sails …] downriver, spends the night at She-Khufu.

[Day 17: casts off from She-Khufu] in the morning,

sails towards Akhet-Khufu; [sails … from] Akhet-Khufu, spends the night at She-Khufu.

[Day 18] […] sails […] spends the night at Tura .

[Day 19]: Inspector Merer] spends the day [with his phyle] hauling stones in Tura [South ?].

Day 20: [Inspector] Mer[er] spends the day with [his phyle] hauling stones in Tura South (?), loads 5 craft, spends the night at Tura.

Day 21: [Inspector] Merer spends the day with his [phyle] loading a transport ship-imu at Tura North, sets sail from Tura in the afternoon.

Day 22: spends the night at Ro-She Khufu. In the morning, sets sail from Ro-She Khufu; sails towards Akhet-Khufu; spends the night at the Chapels of [Akhet] Khufu.

Day 23: The director of 10 Hesi spends the day with his naval section in Ro-She Khufu, because a decision to cast off was taken; spends the night at Ro-She Khufu.

Day 24: Inspector Merer spends the day with his phyle hauling (stones? craft?) with those who are on the register of the Elite, the aper-teams and the noble Ankhhaf, director of Ro-She Khufu.

Day 25: Inspector Merer spends the day with his team hauling stones in Tura, spends the night at Tura North.

[Day 26 …] sails towards […]

That's just a portion if you really want that information do what I did, buy their book. Written by Pierre Tallot, I got the French edition because I was a thirst ball! The English edition is probably available now. Im just saying get into experimenting with other languages, it's the only way to keep your brain growing anyway! I am hoping this book specifically encourages you to do so, when we go to church it's Greek. We are drowning in there, but we struggling to learn how to swim... I challenge you to spend time and learn other cultures, pray in other languages (hoping your at least praying in English), eat some other types of food... That is living! Definitely get back to your roots, but roots grow flowers, bushes and trees... Don't miss the Forest, even the Bible starts in a Garden, **there is all kind plants in a Garden**!

Mdu Ntr
Proto Sinaitic Script
Phoenician
Aramaic, Hebrew, Arabic, Greek
We invented the Papyrus and the writing systems, why would we have even invented papyri without the writings to go on them!

Sound - Mechanical Waves

Script - Ties Mechanical Waves to specific Shapes

The Shapes conjure specific Images in your mind.

Images are internal Light, light that shines in the

Darkness...

Sound becomes Light, Light becomes Flesh.

Friedrich S. Rothschild invented Biosemiotics to investigate this magic between Images and their ability to conjure Sound/Light in your mind! They had access to the hidden knowledge of the Hebrew Alephbeyt and thus the Mdu Ntr. The term biosemiotic was first used by Friedrich S. Rothschild in 1962, but Thomas Sebeok, Thure von Uexküll, Jesper Hoffmeyer and many others have implemented the term and field.

Biosemiotics - from the Greek βίος bios, "life" and σημειωτικός sēmeiōtikos, "observant of signs"... is the field of science composed of semiotics and biology, that studies the prelinguistic meaning-making, biological interpretation processes, production of signs and codes and communication processes in the biological realm.

Ideogram - "ideograph," 1837, from ideo-, here as a combining form of idea, + -gram.

Idea - late 14c., "archetype, concept of a thing in the mind of God," from Latin idea "Platonic idea, archetype," a word in philosophy, the word (Cicero writes it in Greek) and the idea taken from Greek idea "form; the look of a thing; a kind, sort, nature; mode, fashion," in logic, "a class, kind, sort, species," from idein "to see," from PIE *wid-es-ya-, suffixed form of root *weid- "to see."

In Platonic philosophy, "an archetype, or pure immaterial pattern, of which the individual objects in any one natural class are but the imperfect copies, and by participation in which they have their being" [Century Dictionary].

Meaning "mental image or picture" is from 1610s (the Greek word for it was ennoia, originally "act of thinking"), as is the sense "concept of something to be done; concept of what ought to be, differing from what is observed." Sense of "result of thinking" first recorded 1640s.

Idée fixe (1836) is from French, literally "fixed idea." Through Latin the word passed into Dutch, German, Danish as idee, which also is found in English dialects. The philosophical sense has been somewhat further elaborated since 17c. by Descartes, Locke, Berkeley, Hume, Kant. Colloquial big idea (as in what's the ...) is from 1908.

also from late 14c.

Ideagenous - "generating or giving rise to ideas," 1839; see idea + -genous. A word from early psychology, apparently coined by Dr. Thomas Laycock, house surgeon to York County Hospital [Edinburgh Medical and Surgical Journal, vol. lii].

Gram - noun word-forming element, "that which is written or marked," from Greek gramma "that which is drawn; a picture, a drawing; that which is written, a character, an alphabet letter, written letter, piece of writing;" in plural, "letters," also "papers, documents of any kind," also "learning," from stem of graphein "to draw or write" (see -graphy). Some words with it are from Greek compounds, others are modern formations. Alternative -gramme is a French form.

From telegram (1850s) the element was abstracted by 1959 in candygram, a proprietary name in U.S., and thereafter put to wide use as a second element in forming new commercial words, such as Gorillagram (1979), stripagram (1981), and, ultimately, Instagram (2010). The construction violates Greek grammar, as an adverb could not properly form part of a compound noun. An earlier instance was the World War II armed services slang latrinogram "latrine rumor, barracks gossip" (1944).

Phonogram - 1845, "a written symbol or graphic character representing the sound of the human voice," from phono- "sound, voice" + -gram "a writing, recording." From 1879 as "a sound recording produced by a phonograph." Related: Phonogramic.

Pictograph - "pictorial symbol, picture or symbol representing an idea," 1851, from picto-, combining form of Latin pictus "painted," past participle of pingere "to paint" (see paint (v.)) + -graph "something written." First used in reference to American Indian writing. Related: Pictography;

pictographic.

Abstract Sign - are non-representational signs that convey meaning by assignment, without directly representing physical objects, sounds or specific concepts intrinsically.

OSIRIS, AUSAR & WUSIR

Leave to some people and they will claim Osiris, Ausar & Wusir is the trinity. LMAO… He is the central figure in Divinity though. He is the central figure or first king, because he represents Man. Plants and Man, Man as a extension of Plants, something to that effect. Shu is the Hidden one, just like light. 99% of Light is Black to us, not translucent, Black. Close your eyes, that's what you see with no pigment in your eyes. If you have ever been sealed in a soundproof booth, that's what its like to be deaf. We used deaf for not hearing and hearing impaired people, not the same though. We use blind for not seeing and sight impaired people, not the same though. I have healed 'blind' people and given them their eyesight back. That sounds fire because we jump to thinking it means not seeing. I have never done that and don't think it is possible. On the other hand, someone with bad eyes or ears can definitely improve them depending on the cause.

Which brings me to my main thing Diabetes. Osiris was the blue print for Diabetes! The Persians, then the Black Arab Muslims, then the Italians, then all of Europe used sugar as a way to addict, control and enslave the 'Darkies'.

Sugar is addictive and toxic to everyone but... the darker you are, the more it hits and hurts you. That's why liquor is so heavily marketed to you. In Hebrew Likor is to read, and if you want hide something from Black People, put it where? A book!

Mdu Ntr
Proto Sinaitic Script
Phoenician
Aramaic, Hebrew, Arabic, Greek
We invented the Papyrus and the writing systems, why would we have even invented papyri without the writings to go on them!

Sound - Mechanical Waves

Script - Ties Mechanical Waves to specific Shapes

The Shapes conjure specific Images in your mind.

Images are internal Light, light that shines in the Darkness...

Sound becomes Light, Light becomes Flesh.

Friedrich S. Rothschild invented Biosemiotics to investigate this magic between Images and their ability to conjure Sound/Light in your mind! They had access to the hidden knowledge of the Hebrew Alephbeyt and thus the Mdu Ntr. The term biosemiotic was first used by Friedrich S. Rothschild in 1962, but Thomas Sebeok, Thure von Uexküll, Jesper Hoffmeyer and many others have implemented the term and field.

Biosemiotics - from the Greek βίος bios, "life" and σημειωτικός sēmeiōtikos, "observant of signs"... is the field of science composed of semiotics and biology, that studies the prelinguistic meaning-making, biological interpretation processes, production of signs and codes and communication processes in the biological realm.

Ideogram - "ideograph," 1837, from ideo-, here as a combining form of idea, + -gram.

Idea - late 14c., "archetype, concept of a thing in the mind of God," from Latin idea "Platonic idea, archetype," a word in philosophy, the word (Cicero writes it in Greek) and the idea taken from Greek idea "form; the look of a thing; a kind, sort, nature; mode, fashion," in logic, "a class, kind, sort, species," from idein "to see," from PIE *wid-es-ya-, suffixed form of root *weid- "to see."
In Platonic philosophy, "an archetype, or pure immaterial pattern, of which the individual objects in any one natural class are but the imperfect copies, and by participation in which they have their

being" [Century Dictionary].

Meaning "mental image or picture" is from 1610s (the Greek word for it was ennoia, originally "act of thinking"), as is the sense "concept of something to be done; concept of what ought to be, differing from what is observed." Sense of "result of thinking" first recorded 1640s.

Idée fixe (1836) is from French, literally "fixed idea." Through Latin the word passed into Dutch, German, Danish as idee, which also is found in English dialects. The philosophical sense has been somewhat further elaborated since 17c. by Descartes, Locke, Berkeley, Hume, Kant. Colloquial big idea (as in what's the ...) is from 1908.

also from late 14c.

Ideagenous - "generating or giving rise to ideas," 1839; see idea + -genous. A word from early psychology, apparently coined by Dr. Thomas Laycock, house surgeon to York County Hospital [Edinburgh Medical and Surgical Journal, vol. lii].

Gram - noun word-forming element, "that which is written or marked," from Greek gramma "that which is drawn; a picture, a drawing; that which is written, a character, an alphabet letter, written letter, piece of writing;" in plural, "letters," also "papers, documents of any kind," also "learning," from stem of graphein "to draw or write" (see -graphy). Some words with it are from Greek compounds, others are modern formations. Alternative -gramme is a French form.

From telegram (1850s) the element was abstracted by 1959 in candygram, a proprietary name in U.S., and thereafter put to wide use as a second element in forming new commercial words, such as Gorillagram (1979), stripagram (1981), and, ultimately, Instagram (2010). The construction violates Greek grammar, as an adverb could not properly form part of a compound noun. An earlier instance was the World War II armed services slang latrinogram "latrine rumor, barracks gossip" (1944).

Phonogram - 1845, "a written symbol or graphic character representing the sound of the human voice," from phono- "sound, voice" + -gram "a writing, recording." From 1879 as "a sound recording produced by a phonograph." Related: Phonogramic.

Pictograph - "pictorial symbol, picture or symbol representing an idea," 1851, from picto-, combining form of Latin pictus "painted," past participle of pingere "to paint" (see paint (v.)) + -graph "something written." First used in reference to American Indian writing. Related: Pictography; pictographic.

Abstract Sign - are non-representational signs that convey meaning by assignment, without directly representing physical objects, sounds or specific concepts intrinsically.

We invented the Papyrus and the writing systems, why would we have even invented papyri without the writings to go on them!?...

We are globally the dumbest though, like overall we perform the worst in school. There should be no excuses! We should be killing it in school globally, like the Chinese and kids from India. There is of course no culture where everyone is perfect but... We looking crazy right now! Shu, Osiris, Muhammad all of them are turning over in the figurative graves right now!!! Like how Swaye?

We invented Treeless Paper, the writing tools and language, effectively Language Arts should be the study of Mdu Ntr. Then how all other languages branch off that tree, Racism has the whole world in darkness. The race problem - going from god is white and gods children are white to color doesn't matter... you even learn that Europe is a continent...its NOT, its a small group of countries!!! If you tell a school teacher that, they will argue that, then say it doesn't matter.... SMDH... Truth is for them it doesn't matter because 8 billion minds are already colonized...

<u>AS A BIBLE PERSON, I BELIEVE IN THE ONE RACE IDEOLOGY, THE HUMAN RACE. I DO BELIEVE THAT THE DARKER YOU ARE, THE MORE GENETIC INFORMATION YOU HOLD. I THINK THIS IS THE PURPOSE OF THE 'GOD'S CHILDREN REFERENCES. I THINK GOD SAVES HUMANITY BY</u>

<u>SAVING THOSE WITH THE GREATEST GENETIC DIVERSITY. THE GLOBE IS LOSING GENETIC INFORMATION</u>.

Human Genetic Diversity is actually quite low compared to many other species. This is because of a genetic bottleneck in our relatively recent past, when our species was very nearly wiped out. So all modern humans stem from a very, very small population that lived perhaps 900,000-800,000 years ago or just a long time ago (so we aren't debating when the flood/ice age blah blah). The Devil is attempting to create a synthetic Genetic Bottleneck!!! Pushing black people into TransCulture which is a cool way to say sterilized and promoting abortions to the young black moms…

Anyway I am getting way off topic, Wusir & Diabetes.

Deuteronomy 32

8 When the Most High divided to the nations their inheritance, when he separated the sons of Adam, he set the bounds of the people according to the number of the children of Israel.

9 For the Lord's portion is his people; Jacob is the lot of his inheritance.

10 He found him in a desert land, and in the waste howling wilderness; he led him about, he instructed him, he kept him as the apple of his eye.

11 As an eagle stirreth up her nest, fluttereth over her young, spreadeth abroad her wings, taketh them, beareth them on her wings:

12 So the Lord alone did lead him, and there was no strange god with him.

The Bible is a book based on Genetics, to preserve genetics, the wealth and treasures are genetic. There is definitely a few dollars up in there, but that's not God's thing. Chasing endless money is Devil's thing, we have discussed abundance already though. It's just having a lil more than you need to accomplish your earthly Job. Diabetes! LOL… It's so easy for me to get off track.

Osiris was the blue print for Diabetes! The Persians, then the Black Arab Muslims, then the Italians, then all of Europe used sugar as a way to addict, control and enslave the 'Darkies'.

<u>Osiris Blood as Wine</u> (fermented Fruit Sugar). The text book definition of Diabetes (at least in people mind).

<u>Osiris died sealed in a Chess</u> (Chest, Heart Disease). The Heart is the point of attack for Diabetes, and a clogged Heart bars you spiritually from the afterlife. You can't travel through the Heart to reach the "Cross"… You may not even have anything to put on the scale lmao! Imagine folks with fake hearts, if the get to the 'CrossRoad' and they like where is your

Heart? You probably would've just rathered to die, than get a fake heart.

<u>12 Gates of the underworld of Osiris</u> match the 12 gates of the Heart. Don't laugh, the Bible does not break tradition from the focus on your Heart. We literally found the cause, cure and trigger of Death from Heart disease in the Bible! Go get the Speak it into Existence and Observer Effect books, please read &/or reread them.

The Perfect Black physically means Sugar was his kryptonite. You see black people have more type 2b fast twitch muscle, this is the genetic trick, the chink in the armor. This creates the higher susceptibility to Diabetes, Cancer and Heart Disease.

This is also means a preference to Cytochrome 1 for energy production. This also means more Opioid receptors and a stronger Dopamine cascade. Keep going? Larger noses and smaller lungs, tighter cytochromes along the electron transport chain. A higher potential for anabolic hormones (greater crippling effect of stress). The opps caught Osiris slipping with a big fat meal, the 'itis'.

I know there will always be skeptics but remember, you have to ask yourself, how did the Kemetiyu know the speed of Light? How did they know the secret of 137? The Pyramid is not only 137 meters high, 137 is encoded in Shu's Chamber. How did they know that the spot on the Giza plateau was the center of Earth's

Land Mass without a airplane? This is why they want to attribute the Pyramids to Aliens (Demons). Please read the PHD book and the Horus/Set Transaction book.

Inside the 'Kings' Chamber, there is a 'empty' coffin. It's not empty because we know Shu is in it, but for conversation sake… The 'empty' Oblong Square, is the measurement for the room. You can fit exactly 137 Oblong Squares of that exact size, into that room. That means the visible 1, is one out of 137 or 1/137th the room size, get it? Shu's Chamber, the measurement of the end wall diagonally, the length of the chamber and the cubic diagonal are in the exact relationship of 3, 4 and 5. Also, when half of Shu's Chamber width (103.0329+ Pyramid inches, denoted by ½W below) is taken as a unit of measurement, then the other measurements of the chamber are proportionately related via the multiplication of square roots, as follows:

½W x square root of 4 equals the width
½W x square root of 5 equals the height
½W x square root of 9 equals the end diagonal
½W x square root of 16 equals the length
½W x square root of 20 equals the floor diagonal
½W x square root of 21 equals the side diagonal
½W x square root of 25 equals the cubic diagonal
Totaling 100

That further lets you know who's chamber that is,

God. My point is, exploring the inside of the human body, is relatively easy, as opposed to all them complicated measurements and numbers. The point is, the science that was masquerading as religion, is the key to health and protecting your gift, your flesh and breath. 38 is one of them numbers too, you know the sublime mathematics of diabetic arithmetic and there are 38 pyramids in Kemet, just saying… You know Job 38 talk that radio wave talk…

Anyway…

The Bible though…

The breadcrumbs are everywhere, you are the Israelites, yes, you. The Egyptians & Israelites were made up at knife point, those tricky old priests left bread crumbs though. The Name Mizraim, this name does not mean Egypt. The name refers to a slick slang and the name of the Tribe, or at least the modern monicker.

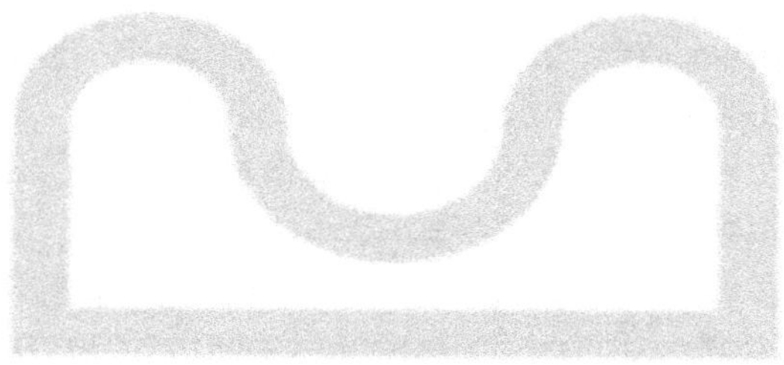

The symbol above or it should be above, printing be 'killin' my books, the Amazon Kindle thing just be re-arranging my stuff… Anyway that symbol is the symbol for mountain, Djew. Djew is the word for mountain, Mount Sinai or Mount Kilimanjaro would be different Djews, get it?

Now the book cover make sense? Mountain Djew? Yeah crazy, giving us diabetes and **troll**ing at the same time! The thing here is the word Mizraim does not mean Egypt it is a code, it's a reference to the Pyramids, the man made Mountains.

Easton's Bible Dictionary - Mizraim (Quoted in the Blue Letter Bible)
Mizraim [N] [H]
the <u>dual form of matzor</u>, meaning a "**mound**" or "fortress," the name of a people descended from Ham (Genesis 10:6 Genesis 10:13 ; 1 Chronicles 1:8 1 Chronicles 1:11). It was the name generally given by the Hebrews to the land of Egypt (q.v.), and may denote the two Egypts, the Upper and the Lower. The modern Arabic name for Egypt is Muzr.

McClintock and Strong Biblical Cyclopedia

Miz'raim (Heb. Mitsra'yim, מִצְרַיִם, if of Heb. origin, meaning two mounds or fortresses, SEE MAZOR, but the word is, perhaps, of foreign [Egyptian or even Arabic] derivation; Sept. Μεσραΐνν; but usually in all the versions, "Egypt" or "Egyptians"), the name by which the Hebrews generally designated Egypt, apparently' from its having been peopled by Mizraim, the second son of Ham (Ge 10:6,13). B.C. post 2513. SEE ABEL- MIZRAIM.

Do you see what I am saying, I have said it in 1000 ways now, the Bible is clearly telling us that, the Israelites & the Egyptians, are the Kemetiyu (Kemetyu). PeriodT. The Djews are the children of Kemet, the Land of the Great Pyramid.

A couple things to note here, the Pyramid, Shu and the Was Sceptre, mean to rise. The Pyramid is the place of rising, the Was Scepter was the tool for rising and Shu was the God of Rising (like heat). In the same pocket as Pharaoh, Egypt and the Nile... Pyramid is a Greek word! There are definitely no Greek Pyramids! Pyramids are called Mir or Mer, means "place of ascent" or "place of rising". The two main theories about the use of the Mir is that it is either a tomb or place to transform post mortem. I disagree, my theory is it is a place to transform the Gods into the flesh. The radio broadcasting of God basically, I know that sounds crazy, but I am cool with it. I firmly believe this is how 'Moses' got the "HeadStones" of the Law, from the electrified mountain... but we discussed that right? Go read &/or reread the Electrician's Prayer Manual & the Electrician's Radio Anatomy Manual. You might as well pull out the Book of Shu too...

Isaiah 19

19 In that day shall there be an altar to the Lord in the midst of the land of Egypt, and a pillar at the border thereof to the Lord.

The point is we need to be alignment spiritually, **<u>WHICH IS THROUGH THE FLESH</u>**!

We have special flesh as Eumelanin dominant people, it is the same color as the Sun. Yes this may be crazy sounding, I am not talking about yellow, redbone or light skinned people either. I am talking brown to black people. Just like the sun, our skin is a impossible color.

Impossible Colors - colors that do not appear in ordinary visual functioning. While some such colors have no basis in reality, phenomena such as cone cell fatigue enable colors to be perceived in certain circumstances that would not be otherwise. The color opponent process is a color theory that states that the human visual system interprets information about color by processing signals from cone and rod cells in an antagonistic manner. The three types of cone cells have some overlap in the wavelengths of light to which they respond, so it is more efficient for the visual system to record differences between the responses of cones, rather than each type of cone's individual response. The opponent color theory suggests that there are three opponent channels:

- Red versus green
- Blue versus orange
- Black versus white (this is achromatic and detects light–dark variation or luminance)

When confront with a specific red/green combination your eyes process them together as Brown. This science is still a hot debate, I mean how can you verify colors you can't see? It's almost like the double slit experiment plays a role, or at least our mind, depth and type of eye pigment... The impossible color thing is crazy, we have that going

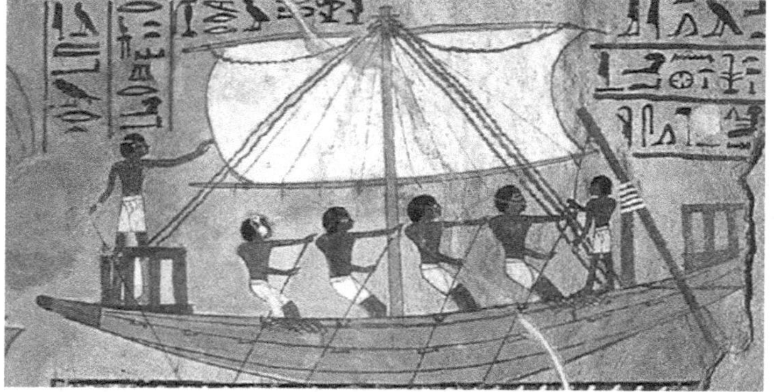

on though. This is why the 'Satanist Alien' people are trying to disguise potential human experimentation, to develop synthetic melanins as "alien research"! This is the same being done with the Olmecs, the problem is the same as in Mizraim, the Stone Work. These are Master Masons beyond our wildest dreams!

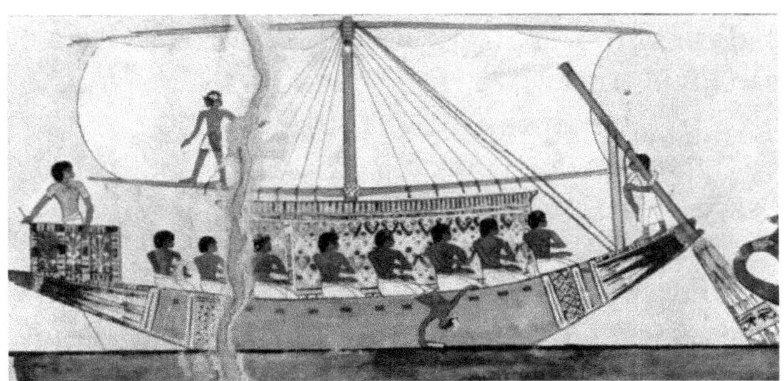

We had boats of all sizes and honestly you didn't really need much, just to catch the wave. The Canary Currents will get from West Africa to America in 2-4 weeks, no problems. This is how we popped up around 1600 bc, the proof is the Masonry. Unmatched.

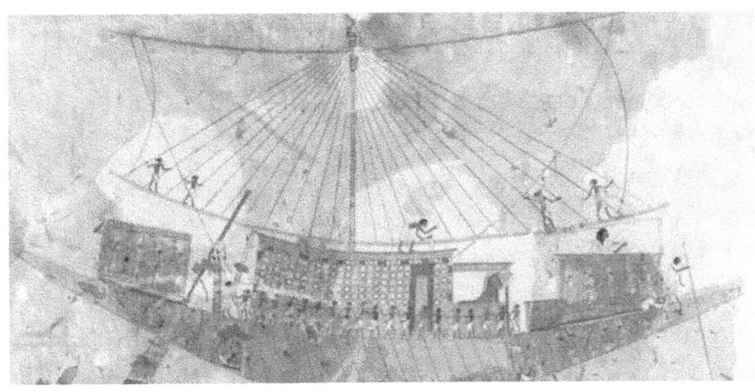

Brief Timeline of Ancient Kemet
Predynastic (ca. 4300-3000 B.C.E.)

Naqada I (Amratian) (ca. 4300 - 3600 B.C.E.)
Naqada II (Gerzean) (ca. 3600 - 3150 B.C.E.)
Naqada III (Semainean) (ca. 3150 - 3000 B.C.E.)
Early Dynastic (ca. 3000 - 2675 B.C.E.)
Dynasty 1 (ca. 3000 - 2800 B.C.E.)
Dynasty 2 (ca. 2800 - 2675 B.C.E.)
Old Kingdom (ca. 2675 - 2130 B.C.E)
Dynasty 3 (ca. 2675 - 2625 B.C.E.)
Dynasty 4 (ca. 2625 - 2500 B.C.E)
Dynasty 5 (ca. 2500 - 2350 B.C.E.)
Dynasty 6 (ca. 2350 - 2710 B.C.E)
Dynasties 7-8 (ca. 2170 - 2130 B.C.E.)
First Intermediate Period (ca. 2130 - 1980 B.C.E.)
Dynasties 9-10 (ca. 2130 - 1970 B.C.E.)
Dynasty 11, Part I (ca. 2081 - 1980 B.C.E.)
Middle Kingdom (ca. 1980 - 1630 B.C.E.)
Dynasty 11, Part II (ca. 1980 - 1938 B.C.E)
Dynasty 12 (ca. 1938 - 1759 B.C.E.)
Dynasty 13 (ca. 1759 - after 1630 B.C.E.)
Dynasty 14 (dates uncertain, but contemporary with later Dynasty 13)
Second Intermediate period (ca. 1630 - 1539/1523 B.C.E)
Dynasty 15 (ca. 1630 - 1523 B.C.E.)
Dynasty 16 (dates unknown: minor Hyksos rulers, contemporary with Dynasty 15)
Dynasty 17 (ca. 1630 - 1539 B.C.E.)
NEW KINGDOM (ca. 1539 - 1075 B.C.E.)
Dynasty 18 (ca. 1539 - 1292 B.C.E.)
Dynasty 19 (ca. 1292 - 1190 B.C.E.)

Dynasty 20 (ca. 1190 - 1075 B.C.E.)
THIRD INTERMEDIATE PERIOD (ca. 1075 - 656 B.C.E.)
Dynasty 21 (ca. 1075 - 945 B.C.E.)
Dynasty 22 (ca. 945 - 712 B.C.E.)
Dynasty 23 (ca. 838 - 712 B.C.E.)
Dynasty 24 (ca. 727 - 712 B.C.E.)
Dynasty 25 (ca. 760 - 656 B.C.E.)
LATE PERIOD (ca. 664 - 332 B.C.E.)
Dynasty 26 (ca. 664 - 525 B.C.E.)
Dynasty 27 (ca. 525 - 404 B.C.E.)
Dynasty 28 (ca. 404 - 399 B.C.E.)
Dynasty 29 (ca. 399 - 380 B.C.E.)
Dynasty 30 (ca. 380 - 343 B.C.E.)
Dynasty 31 (ca. 343 - 332 B.C.E.)
MACEDONIAN PERIOD (ca. 332 - 305 B.C.E.)
Alexander the Great and his successors
PTOLEMAIC DYNASTY (ca. 305 - 30 B.C.E.)
Ptolemy I and ending with Cleopatra VII
ROMAN and BYZANTINE EMPIRE (ca. 30 B.C.E. - 642 C.E.)
Beginning with Augustus Caesar

I put this here because my theory is that when the Hyksos took over Kemet, people abandoned ship! The time that the first Hyksos take power is when the first proof of Olmecs is dated to. There is plenty of evidence about genetics, head shapes, writing systems etc... linking the Olemcs to the Kemetyu, the thing is I never saw a real reason to bounce from Kemet. A little bit of digging and boom, cause I was thinking the same thing if Kamala Harris got in office. Luckily we got Trump, just saying... I figured something had to go crazy, and sure enough the time periods are a match.

Please don't fail to see that these are Mental & Spiritual Health books. We need to get our minds right, I showed the physical damage your Amygdala suffers by worshipping foreign Gods. In the previous books.

I just want you to start praying for the new year and the Holy Days (whichever ones you celebrate). Lets pray, I am trying to tell you that is the trick. You have Ancestors waiting to hear from you!!!! They all didn't make it, but some are around for you.

PRAYER WORK

The Lord's Prayer

Greek/English

"EvloyeeMENee ee vasilehEEah tou PatrOS, kai tou EeOU, kai tou AhyEEou PNEVmatos." (Blessed is the Kingdom of the Father, and of the Son, and of the Holy Spirit.)

"Neen kai ahEE, kai EEs tous eeOnas ton eOnon. AmEEn." (Now and ever and unto ages of ages. Amen.)

"EHtee kai EHtee en eerEEnee tou KeerEEou deheethOmen." (Again and again in peace, let us pray to the Lord.)

"Tess presVEEehs tees ThehoTOkou, SOtare, SOson eeMAS." (Through the prayers of the Theotokos, Savior, save us."

"SOson eemas, Ee-eh ThehOU, o anaSTAS ek nekRON, sallontAS see. Ah-lee-LOO-ee-ah" (Save us, O Son of God, Who art risen from the dead, save us who sing to Thee. Alleluia.)

"AhyeeOs O ThehOs, Ahyeeos Eekeeros, Ahyeeos ATHAnatos, eLEHeeson eeMAS." (Holy God, Holy Mighty, Holy Immortal, have mercy on us.)

"Thoxa PaTREE, keh EEou, keh AyEEou PNEVmahtee." (Glory to the Father, and to the Son, and to the ages of ages."

"KEE-ree-eh eLEHeeson." (Lord, have mercy)

"PaRAskoo KEE-ree-eh." (Grant this, O Lord)

"Kai to PNEVmati sou" (And with thy spirit.)

"THOksa see, kee-ree-eh, THOksa see." (Glory to Thee, O Lord, glory to Thee.)

The Lord's Prayer (Greek)

ΠΑΤΕΡ ΗΜΩΝ Ο ΕΝ ΤΟΙΣ ΟΥΡΑΝΟΙΣ ΑΓΙΑΣΘΗΤΩ ΤΟ ΟΝΟΜΑ ΣΟΥ ΕΛΘΕΤΩ Η ΒΑΣΙΛΕΙΑ ΣΟΥ ΓΕΝΗΘΗΤΩ ΤΟ ΘΕΛΗΜΑ ΣΟΥ, ΩΣ ΕΝ ΟΥΡΑΝΩ ΚΑΙ ΕΠΙ ΤΗΣ ΓΗΣ ΤΟΝ ΑΡΤΟΝ ΗΜΩΝ ΤΟΝ ΕΠΙΟΥΣΙΟΝ ΔΟΣ ΗΜΙΝ ΣΗΜΕΡΟΝ ΚΑΙ ΑΦΕΣ ΗΜΙΝ ΤΑ ΟΦΕΙΛΗΜΑΤΑ ΗΜΩΝ, ΩΣ ΚΑΙ ΗΜΕΙΣ ΑΦΙΕΜΕΝ ΤΟΙΣ ΟΦΕΙΛΕΤΑΙΣ ΗΜΩΝ ΚΑΙ ΜΗ ΕΙΣΕΝΕΓΚΗΣ ΗΜΑΣ ΕΙΣ ΠΕΙΡΑΣΜΟΝ, ΑΛΛΑ ΡΥΣΑΙ ΗΜΑΣ ΑΠΟ ΤΟΥ ΠΟΝΗΡΟΥ. ΑΜΗΝ.

Pater hêmôn ho en toes ouranoes; hagiasthêtô to onoma sou; elthetô hê basileia sou; genêthêtô to thelêma sou, hôs en ouranô, kae epi tês gês. ton arton hêmôn ton epiousion dos hêmin sêmeron; kae aphes hêmin ta opheilêmata hêmôn, hôs kae hêmeis aphiemen toes opheiletaes hêmôn; kae mê eisenenkês hêmas eis peirasmon, alla rhysae hêmas apo tou ponerou. hoti sou estin hê basileia kae hê dynamis kae hê doxa eis tous aeônas; amên.

Our Father who art in heaven
Hallowed be thy name
Thy Kingdom come
Thy will be done
On Earth as it is in Heaven
Give us this day our daily bread
And forgive us our trespasses
As we forgive those who trespass against us
And lead us not into temptation
But deliver us from evil
For thine is the kingdom
And the power, and the glory
For ever and ever
Amen

Egyptian Version - The Egyptian Book of the Dead Spell 125 addressed the weighing of the deceased's heart. Osiris weighs the deceased's heart in a pan, balancing it against the weight of a feather. This is balancing the Magnetism of the Heart vs the

Electricity of the Feather, the Underworld of Wusir vs The Sky of Shu. If the heart is as a **light** as the feather, Ausar pronounces the soul fit for immortality (to join Shu). Spell 125 is said to be the original version of the Lord's Prayer, guarantying that the possessor of the book should be granted access to the afterlife, if his or her "heart" is judged morally as **light,** in respect to the **weight** of the **42 negative confessions** (forerunner to the ten commandments). Those confessions act on that Almond Joy... Below is a comparison of the Spell 125 and ...

Our Father who art in heaven
Hallowed be thy name

Hail gods who dwell in the house of two truths (goddesses). I know you and your names

Thy Kingdom come
Thy will be done
On Earth as it is in Heaven

I have acted according to his will

Give us this day our daily bread

I have given bread to the hungry man and water to the thirsty man, and clothes to the naked man, and a boat to the boatels.
I havemade holy offerings to the gods,
And meals for the dead

Deliver me, protect me, accuse me not in the presence of Osiris.
I am pure of mouth and hands....

And forgive us our trespasses
As we forgive those who trespass against us

Who lives on the entrails of the mighty ones on the day of judgement. Grant that I may come to you,
For I have committed no faults
I have not sinned

And lead us not into temptation
But deliver us from evil

Let no evil come to me from you
Declare me right and true in the presence of Osiris,
Because I have done what is right and true in Egypt...
Deliver me from the god BABA
I have not done evil...

For thine is the kingdom
And the power, and the glory
For ever and ever
Amen

Let me not fall under your slaughter-knives,
And do not bring my wickedness to Osiris, the god you serve.
Amen

Address at arrival at the broad hall of the Two

Goddesses of What is Right,
shielding ________ (say your name) from all forbidden things that he has done, and seeing the faces of the gods.
Words spoken by ________ (say your name):
Hail great god, lord of the place of the Two Goddesses of What is Right.
I have come before you so that you may bring me to see your perfection.
I know you, I know your name,
I know the name of these 42 gods who are with you in this broad court of the Two Goddesses of What is Right,
who live on the henchmen of evil, and eat of their blood
on that day of calculating characters in the presence of Wennefer.
See, your name is He of the two Daughters, he of the two Chants, lord of the Two Goddesses of What is Right,
See, I am come before you, I have brought What is Right to you, I have removed What is Wrong for you.
I have not impoverished the divine herd (people); I have committed no crime in place of What is Right;
I have not known (explored) nothingness; I have not done any evil
I have not made a daily start in labours over what I did (previously);
My name has not reached the office of director of servants;

I have not orphaned the orphan of his goods;
I have not done the abomination of the gods;
I have not slighted a servant to his master;
I have not caused affliction; I have not caused hunger;
I have not caused grief; I have not killed;
I have not harmed the offering-cattle; I have not caused pain for anyone;
I have not reduced the offerings in the temples;
I have not harmed the offering-loaves of the gods;
I have not taken the festival-loaves of the blessed dead;
I have not penetrated the penetrater of a penetrater; I have not masturbated;
I have not reduced the measuring-vessel, I have not reduced the measuring cord;
I have not encroached on the fields; I have not added to the pan of the scales;
I have not tampered with the plumb bob of the scales;
I have not taken milk from the mouths of babes;
I have not concealed herds from their pastures;
I have not snared birds in the thickets (?) of the gods;
I have not caught fish in their pools;
I have not held back water in its time;
I have not dammed a dam at rapid waters;
I have not put out the fire in its moment;
I have not transgressed the days concerning meat offerings;
I have not turned back cattle from the property of a god;
I have not blocked a god in his processions;

I am pure (four times),
my purity is the purity of that great phoenix which is in Henenesut,
because I am indeed that nose of the lord of breath,
who enables all the populace to live, on that day of filling the Sound Eye in Iunu, on month 2 of winter, last day.
I am the one who sees the filling of the Sound Eye in Iunu.
Nothing evil can befall me in this land, in this broad hall of the Two Goddesses of What is Right,
because I know the names of the gods who dwell in it.

Those are probably crazy imperfect, they are right enough for you to get going!

EnQi Prayer
Hail SHU who Created the Heavens & the Earth, Hail Wusir who gave us Pigment.
And there was Electromagnetic Waves, before and beyond our pigment created Light, for which we give thanks.
And there was Mechanical Waves, before and beyond our pigment created Sound, for which we give thanks.
And there is heat, for which we are grateful.
And there is power, for which we are grateful.
Blessed be Tefnuit & Nuit, for giving us a womb made of water.
Blessed be Shu & Geb, who gave us

ElectroMagnetism.
Blessed be Djehuti, who gave us wisdom.
Blessed be Atum-Re, who gave us sight.

We give thanks for the Blessings of Shu.

Blessed are we for cellular E.L.F waves, so our cells can talk to each other.

Blessed are we for long radio waves, which oscillate slowly.

Blessed are we for broadcast waves, for which we educate & communicate with via Djed Pillars natural and handmade.

Blessed are we for short waves, linkers of humankind.

Blessed are we for microwaves, that we may sea better.

Blessed are we for infrared, bearers of nourishing heat and Melatonin.

Blessed are we for visible light, tuned to our waters.

Blessed are we for red, sacred to Set.

Blessed are we for orange (dark yellow there was no orange in Kemet), sacred to the Rising Sun.

Blessed are we for Khenet (yellow), hallowed by Re's gaze.

Blessed are we for sWadj (green), the color of our skin, gift from Wusir.

Blessed are we for Khesbedj (lazuli Blue), for its hydrogen line and recycling Vitamin A.

Blessed are we for Irtyu (indigo), which tricks us by looking mefkhat (turquoise) sometime.

Blessed are we for violet, flourishing with energy.

Blessed are we for ultraviolet, which creates Melanin & Vitamin D.

Blessed are we for X rays, sacred to stone, that we may sea better.

Blessed are we for the gamma, dangerously high vibrations.

We give thanks for the Geniuses Tesla, Mesmer, Swan, Brush, Planck, Einstein, Thomas, Heaviside, Steinmetz, West, Brown (a sister), Easley (a sister), Morgan (Black Edison), Latimer, Sampson, Russell, Turner, Sebi, Becker and others that re-membered the body of Shu-Amun for us.

In light of Light and Sound, in light of Electromagnetic Waves, Mechanical Waves and the Holy Trinity, Amen!

Khem/Black - has all the magic, all the lights not visible to the human eye are in the Black part of the Spectrum. Clear symbolizes empty, black symbolize abundance beyond what your eyes can see! Cup runneth over, is a reference to the blood of Osiris flooding with black soil... Khem.Black (Ancient Egyptian name "kem") was the color of the life-giving silt left by the Nile inundation, which gave rise to the Ancient Egyptian name for the country: "kemet" – the black land.

Silver (also known by the name "hedj," but written with the determinative for precious metal) represented the color of the sun at dawn, and the moon, and stars.

White (Ancient Egyptian name "hedj") was the color of purity, sacredness, cleanliness and simplicity.

Blue (Ancient Egyptian name "irtyu") was the color of the heavens, the dominion of the gods, as well as the color of water, Ancient Egyptians favored semi-precious stones such as azurite (Ancient Egyptian name "tefer'" and lapis lazuli (Ancient Egyptian name "khesbedj," imported at great cost across the Sinai Desert... Blue was used for the hair of gods (specifically lapis lazuli, or the darkest of Egyptian blues) and for the face of the god Amun...

Green (Ancient Egyptian name "wahdj'"was the color of fresh growth, vegetation, new life and resurrection (the latter along with the color black). The hieroglyph for green is a papyrus stem and frond. Green was the color of the "Eye of Horus," or "Wedjat," which had healing and protective powers, and so the color also represented well-being. To do "green things" was to do behave in a positive, life-affirming manner. When written with the **determinative** for minerals (three grains of sand) "wahdj" becomes the word for malachite, a color which represented joy.

Turquoise (Ancient Egyptian name "mefkhat"), a particularly valued green-blue stone from the Sinai, also represented joy, as well as the color of the sun's rays at dawn.

Yellow (Ancient Egyptian name "khenet") was the color of women's skin, as well as the skin of people who lived near the Mediterranean - Libyans, Bedouin, Syrians and Hittites.

Gold (Ancient Egyptian name "newb") represented the flesh of the gods and was used for anything which was considered eternal or indestructible. (Gold was used on a sarcophagus, for example, because the pharaoh had become a god.)

Red (Ancient Egyptian name "deshr") was primarily the color of chaos and disorder – the color of the desert (Ancient Egyptian name "deshret," the red land) which was considered the opposite of the fertile black land ("kemet"). Red was also the color of destructive fire and fury and was used to represent something dangerous, red ochre or hematite for red; yellow ochre for yellow; Egyptian blue was a synthetic pigment created mainly from copper silica and calcium; green from malachite (a natural copper ore) or, then, from a paste manufactured by mixing oxides of copper and iron with silica and calcium; and black was made of carbon compounds (soot, ground charcoal, and animal bones).

Mdu Ntr
Proto Sinaitic Script
Phoenician
Aramaic, Hebrew, Arabic, Greek
We invented the Papyrus and the writing systems,

why would we have even invented papyri without the writings to go on them!

Sound - Mechanical Waves

Script - Ties Mechanical Waves to specific Shapes

The Shapes conjure specific Images in your mind.

Images are internal Light, light that shines in the Darkness...

Sound becomes Light, Light becomes Flesh.

Friedrich S. Rothschild invented Biosemiotics to investigate this magic between Images and their ability to conjure Sound/Light in your mind! They had access to the hidden knowledge of the Hebrew Alephbeyt and thus the Mdu Ntr. The term biosemiotic was first used by Friedrich S. Rothschild in 1962, but Thomas Sebeok, Thure von Uexküll, Jesper Hoffmeyer and many others have implemented the term and field.

Biosemiotics - from the Greek βίος bios, "life" and σημειωτικός sēmeiōtikos, "observant of signs"... is the field of science composed of semiotics and biology, that studies the prelinguistic meaning-making, biological interpretation processes, production of signs and codes and communication processes in the biological realm.

Ideogram - "ideograph," 1837, from ideo-, here as a combining form of idea, + -gram.

Idea - late 14c., "archetype, concept of a thing in the mind of God," from Latin idea "Platonic idea, archetype," a word in philosophy, the word (Cicero writes it in Greek) and the idea taken from Greek idea "form; the look of a thing; a kind, sort, nature; mode, fashion," in logic, "a class, kind, sort, species," from idein "to see," from PIE *wid-es-ya-, suffixed form of root *weid- "to see."

In Platonic philosophy, "an archetype, or pure immaterial pattern, of which the individual objects in any one natural class are but the imperfect copies, and by participation in which they have their being" [Century Dictionary].

Meaning "mental image or picture" is from 1610s (the Greek word for it was ennoia, originally "act of thinking"), as is the sense "concept of something to be done; concept of what ought to be, differing from what is observed." Sense of "result of thinking" first recorded 1640s.

Idée fixe (1836) is from French, literally "fixed idea." Through Latin the word passed into Dutch, German, Danish as idee, which also is found in English dialects. The philosophical sense has been somewhat further elaborated since 17c. by Descartes, Locke, Berkeley, Hume, Kant. Colloquial big idea (as in what's the ...) is from 1908.

also from late 14c.

Ideagenous - "generating or giving rise to ideas," 1839; see idea + -genous. A word from early psychology, apparently coined by Dr. Thomas Laycock, house surgeon to York County Hospital [Edinburgh Medical and Surgical Journal, vol. lii].

Gram - noun word-forming element, "that which is written or marked," from Greek gramma "that which is drawn; a picture, a drawing; that which is written, a character, an alphabet letter, written letter, piece of writing;" in plural, "letters," also "papers, documents of any kind," also "learning," from stem of graphein "to draw or write" (see -graphy). Some words with it are from Greek compounds, others are modern formations. Alternative -gramme is a French form.
From telegram (1850s) the element was abstracted by 1959 in candygram, a proprietary name in U.S., and thereafter put to wide use as a second element in forming new commercial words, such as Gorillagram (1979), stripagram (1981), and, ultimately, Instagram (2010). The construction violates Greek grammar, as an adverb could not properly form part of a compound noun. An earlier instance was the World War II armed services slang latrinogram "latrine rumor, barracks gossip" (1944).

Phonogram - 1845, "a written symbol or graphic character representing the sound of the human voice," from phono- "sound, voice" + -gram "a writing, recording." From 1879 as "a sound recording produced by a phonograph." Related: Phonogramic.

Pictograph - "pictorial symbol, picture or symbol representing an idea," 1851, from picto-, combining form of Latin pictus "painted," past participle of pingere "to paint" (see paint (v.)) + -graph "something written." First used in reference to American Indian writing. Related: Pictography; pictographic.

Abstract Sign - are non-representational signs that convey meaning by assignment, without directly representing physical objects, sounds or specific concepts intrinsically.

Mdu Ntr
Proto Sinaitic Script
Phoenician
Aramaic, Hebrew, Arabic, Greek
We invented the Papyrus and the writing systems, why would we have even invented papyri without the writings to go on them!

Sound - Mechanical Waves

Script - Ties Mechanical Waves to specific Shapes

The Shapes conjure specific Images in your mind.

Images are internal Light, light that shines in the Darkness...

Sound becomes Light, Light becomes Flesh.

So when all prayers end in Amen, it is directed to the Hidden one, God of the Wind, Breath & Light. Shu and Amun are one in the same (in my research), Amun was used in countries where Shu was not. The Ennead was in Heliopolis (Iunu) and the Ogdoad was in Hermopolis (Khmunu). The 9 Gods of creation vs the 8 Gods + a hidden God of creation.

TaNeter - Great Lakes origin of the Hapi River (mount Kilimanjaro)
TaSeti - Nubia
TaMeri - Kemet (Tawy was like the slang version like 'tha house')

This is why science traces Haplotypes from south Africa, Greece learned from Egypt, Europe is just copying and expounding on Greece.

The word Hieroglyph is Greek... It means sacred engravings, divine engravings or God's engravings! Mdu Ntr is the Word of God **in the Bible**.

You can tap into Ramesses the 2nd Prayer, the first recorded Monotheistic Prayer in History, before Akhenaten &/or Moses. This is in the battle for Kadesh! This battle is between the Khemites and the Hittites... This seals the Deal!!! The Israelites have to be either the Khemites or Hittites in history! This is the southern border of Israel/Canaan/Judah...

The Tribe of Shu or the Tribe of the DJews, the people who made the Mountains!!! Yep, you have been trolled all these years with the soda play on it, just to let you know in a devilish way, once you find out… They been knew, hid it and used it against you! Mountain Djew! Crazy because I have very warm memories, from my childhood with Mountain 'DJew' in there, it was my favorite at one point. I mean my father gave me 3 options, Water, Tropican Orange Juice or Mountain DJou soda!

Sa-Hut en-ek, it-en Amen-Ra

I call to you, Oh our father Amun-Ra

Nakhet en senedj mehu neferu

We are surrounded by unfamiliar enemies with hostile intentions

Sutenet nebwet senedj ten

These nations have come together against us

Peru ek nebet nekh Kamet nefer

To harm Khemites and steal our riches

Wekh djet khef ni seru kher

We are alone with no one by our side

Sehut t'j khef lunu-Waset

My cry reaches Waset (Thebes)

Sedjer sekhet senet khef ser-ek

And I hear your footsteps coming to help us

Dewaut en-ek Amen-Ra neb pet ta

Glory to you Oh Amun-Ra Master of the Universe

The secret Ceremony of Rabbi's to speak the name of God you are never supposed to say...

Zechariah 14:9

And the Lord shall be king over all the earth: in that day shall there be one Lord, and his name one.

In Hebrew is the secret....

"And his name" in hebrew is pronounced Ooo Shu Mo!!!

ט וְהָיָה יְהוָה לְמֶלֶךְ עַל-כָּל-הָאָרֶץ; בַּיּוֹם הַהוּא, יִהְיֶה יְהוָה אֶחָד--וּשְׁמוֹ אֶחָד.

Ooo Shu Mo = וּשְׁמוֹ

"Yahweh" is not his name it is a attribute like the hidden one, invisible one, air, wind etc... The Phoenician šin letter expressed the continuants of two Proto-Semitic phonemes, and may have been based on a pictogram of a tooth (in modern Hebrew shen). The Encyclopaedia Judaica, 1972, records that it originally represented a composite bow. The Shen in the Hebrew alephbeyt is like a W... It makes a SH sound, not a wuh... The thing is even in

English, the Double U is wild, it's the only letter with two syllables. The double u is also a golden spiral, keeping it 100 (pun intended).

Shu is God that came in the Flesh as Wusir.

Yehova - I am that I am, I be, I exist etc…

Listen the secret ceremony is said to be done standing in water, why? What is the sound of running water in nature? Sshhuuuuu!!! Just like white noise, white noise is the equal reception of unlimited frequencies…. Ssshhhhuuuuu!!! A small body of water is called a sound. Fire burning, electricity doing it's thing…. Shh!

I type too fast sometimes, I want to drop 1 last jewel on you, the name of God that you can't say. The name you can't say is transmitted my secret ritual, mouth to ear, standing in water at least ankle high.

The key is Zechariah 14:9, well you got it I think…

Generating clean electricity with chicken feathers

Turning unused waste from food production into clean energy.
By
Amit Malewar
23 Oct, 2023

Go read that article…. Lmao…

Sidebar...

A jar of almonds was found in Tutankhamen's tomb. Almonds were also among the best products of the land sent by Jacob to the man in Egypt (Genesis 43:11).

DR.ENQI

Raw Herbal Compounds
PRODUCT GUIDE

Detox Kit:

Kemeluminescence -
NRF2, YEAST, FUNGUS, FAT SUPPORT;
Bladderwrack, Yarrow, Cascara Sagrada, Moss, Happy Tree, Madagascar, Periwinkle, Mayapple, Pacific Yew, Cloves, Amla, Coriander, Black Walnut, Kelp, White Pine Bark, Horny Goat Weed, Milk Thistle, Tribulus, Bitter Melon, Chaste Berry, African Pygeum, Cinnamon, Gynesylvestre, Hemp, Pau D Arco, African Bird Pepper, Cinchona Bark, Chinese Senega Root, Biden Pilosa, Houttuynia, Licorice, Skullcap, Scute Root, Ginseng, Rehmania, Er Bu Shir Tao, Bugleweed
Swadj Momatomix -
Marrow & Electromagnetism Support / Rich in Hydrogen, Phosphorus, Aromatic Amino Acid
Phosphorus, Nettles, Wild Lettuce, Hydrogen, Plant Enzyme, &Alkaloid+ MATRIX

Antiviral Kit -

Antiviral
Antifungal
Antibacterial
mtDNA Protector
The most comprehensive organic antiviral kit ever assembled to fight viral infection and improve recovery

Antivirals -
Exogenous & Endogenous Pathogen Support
Cilantro, Celery, Chaparral, Olive Leaf, Oregano Leaf, Black Walnut, Lysine, Tyrosine, Thyme, Cleavers, Hyssop, Bladderwrack, Ginger

Antiviral Nutrient -
Pathogen Suppression Support
Manganese, Rosemary, Hydrangea, Bilberry, Rhizome Rei

Antiviral Oil -
Immunglobulin & Antibody Support
Oregano, Peppermint, Tea Tree, Cinnamon, Hyssop, Thyme, Clove, Ginger

Calcium -
Muscle & Bone Support
Blood Pressure, Insulin Control, Nerve Function, Muscle Contraction
Kelp, Calcium, Sesame, Cloves

Chromium & Vanadium -

Glucose Tolerance Factor & Eyesight Support
Fat Loss , Insulin Metabolism , Hydration , Muscle Integrity , Energy
Chromium, Fenugreek, Vanadium, Bitter Melon, Gymnema Sylvestre

Copper -
Pigment System Support
Cardiovascular Key, Heart Beat Nutrient, White Blood Cell Reg
Copper, Cilantro, Cloves, Milk Thistle

Iron -
Heme & Magnetism Support
Electron Circulation, Digestive System, Thermogenesis, Brain Power
Iron, Yellow Dock, Stinging Nettles, Chaparral

Magnesium -
Energy & Light Metabolism Support
Muscle Function, Energy, Builds ; Proteins/ Enzymes/ Hormones , DNA Repair
Blue Vervain, Burdock, Parsley, Magnesium

Muscle Drip -
Children/Adults Multivitamin & Bone Tendon Compound
Blood Oxygen, Breakdown Lactic Acid, Builds Blood Cells Faster, Cleans Lymphatic System
Elderberries, Cherries, Sea Moss, Stinging Nettles, Horsetail, Lily of the Valley, Bladderwrack, Bromide,

Melatonin, Phosphorus, Boron, Calcium, Strontium

Muscle Plants -
Children + Adults Multivitamin & Muscle/Joint Compound
Gout, Autography, Enhanced Healing, Arthritis, Remove Stones
Elderberries, Cherries, Bugleweed, Hombre Grande, Blue Vervain, Chaparral, Ginseng, Rhodiola, Boswellia, Eluethero, Melatonin, Phosphorus, Magnesium

Selenium -
Immune Plasma Support
Thyroid Health, Cancer Suppression, Mental Health, Tumor Suppression
Selenium, Burdock, Bladderwrack, Sarsaparilla

Swadj Momatomix -
Marrow & Electromagnetism Support / Rich in Hydrogen, Phosphorus, Aromatic Amino Acid
Phosphorus, Nettles, Wild Lettuce, Hydrogen, Plant Enzyme, &Alkaloid+ MATRIX

Zinc -
Skin & Enzyme Support
Anabolic Boost, Immune System Nutrient, Stem Cell Health, Gene Support
Rosemary, Chlorella, Sage, Zinc

Watermelanin -
Nootropic, Dopamine, Muscle Recovery, Nourish

Your Pineal Gland, DMT Support
Raw Organic Non-GMO Black Watermelon Seeds
Lupulin

Anabolic Hormone Help -
Anabolic Hormones, AMPK & Circadian Support
Jiaogulan, Wild Lettuce, Tribulus, Longjack, Maca &
Pollen Blend

Histonic -
Histone Sirtuin Support
Grape Skin, Resveratrol, Tyrosine Analogue, Japanese
Knotweed

Ocean Steak -
Vegan B12, Carbon, Nucleoside, Protein, Nucleotide,
Omega 3 & Eye Support
Phytoplankton, Duckweed, Chlorella, Purple Laver,
Chondrus Crispus & C60 Lutein, Zeaxanthin, Ocean
Pigment Matrix

Chrondris Crispus -
Structured Water Mucus Membrane Support
Copper, Cilantro, Cloves, Milk Thistle

NON GMO Moringa -
Whole Body Nutrition Support
Raw Organic Non-GMO Moringa

Purple Phaze -
Anti-Aging Longevity Support
FoTi, Pumpkin Seed, NMN, Bhringaraj, Biotin, Silica,
Tyrosine, Yucca, White Willow Bark, French Lilac,

NAD

Every item on this list, every compound is not only from God but works on the skin from the inside out, what we need now is topical.

Topical = Tropical

Batana is Great but it's expensive and incomplete.

Researchers identify 135 new melanin genes responsible for pigmentation

Date: August 11, 2023

Source: University of Oklahoma

Summary: The skin, hair and eye color of more than eight billion humans is determined by the light-absorbing pigment known as melanin. New research has identified 135 new genes associated with pigmentation. Vitamin D and Vitamin A... I told you nature doesn't wait to be discovered before getting to work! Melanin vs Diabetes as a Ministry & Movement isn't waiting around to save lives... We have saving lives and creating thought leaders for 20 years!!! The thing is science just discovered 135 genes for pigment and melanin, how the F@3$ have the been acting as if.... This is why we rely on Nature, God & our Ancestors.

We are teaching the world, showing the world...

#HealingLooksLikeThis

Most people don't know what the process of Healing actually Looks Like!!!

People judge health by how your skin looks, literally your complexion. Your Complex of Ions!

Complexion - the general aspect or character of something; the natural color, texture, and appearance of a person's skin, especially of the face.

complexion (n.)
mid-14c., complexioun, "temperament, natural disposition of body or mind," from Old French complexion, complession "**combination of humors**," hence "temperament, character, make-up," from Latin complexionem (nominative complexio) "combination" (in Late Latin, "physical constitution"), from complexus "surrounding, encompassing," past participle of complecti "to encircle, embrace," in transferred use, "to hold fast, master, comprehend," from com "with, together" (see com-) + plectere "to weave, braid, twine, entwine," from PIE *plek-to-, suffixed form of root *plek- "to plait."
The Middle English sense is from the old medicine notion of bodily constitution or general nature resulting from blending of the four primary qualities (hot, cold, dry, moist) or humors (blood, phlegm, choler, black choler). The specific meaning

"**<u>color or hue of the skin of the face</u>**" developed by mid-15c. In medieval physiology, the color of the face was believed to be caused by the balance of humors in the body and indicate temperament or health. The word rarely is used in the sense of "state of being complex."
also from mid-14c.

Humor - the quality of being amusing or comic, especially as expressed in literature or speech; a mood or state of mind. **Each of the four chief fluids of the body (blood, phlegm, yellow bile (choler), and black bile (melancholy)) that were thought to determine a person's physical and mental qualities** by the relative proportions in which they were present.

humor (n.)
mid-14c., "**fluid or juice of an animal or plant**," from Old North French humour "liquid, dampness; (medical) humor" (Old French humor, umor; Modern French humeur), from Latin umor "body fluid" (also humor, by false association with **humus "earth"**); related to umere "**be wet**, moist," and to uvescere "become wet" (see humid).
In old medicine, "any of the four body fluids" (blood, phlegm, choler, and melancholy or black bile).

*The human body had four humors—blood, phlegm, yellow bile, and black bile—which, in turn, were associated with particular organs. Blood came from the heart, phlegm from the brain, yellow bile from the liver, and black bile from the spleen. Galen and Avicenna attributed certain elemental qualities to each humor. Blood was hot and moist, like air; phlegm was cold and moist, like water; yellow bile was hot and dry, like fire; and black bile was cold and dry, like earth. In effect, the human body was a microcosm of the larger world. [Robert S. Gottfried, "The Black Death," 1983]

Their relative proportions were thought to determine physical condition and state of mind. This gave humor an extended sense of "mood, temporary state of mind" (recorded from 1520s); the sense of "amusing quality, funniness, jocular turn of mind" is first recorded 1680s, probably via sense of "whim, caprice" as determined by state of mind (1560s), which also produced the verb sense of "indulge (someone's) fancy or disposition." Modern French has them as doublets: humeur "disposition, mood, whim;" humour "humor." "The pronunciation of the initial h is only of recent date, and is sometimes omitted ..." [OED].

For aid in distinguishing the various devices that tend to be grouped under "humor," this guide, from Henry W. Fowler ["Modern English Usage," 1926] may be of use:

HUMOR: motive/aim: discovery; province: human nature; method/means: observation; audience: the sympathetic

WIT: motive/aim: throwing light; province: words & ideas; method/means: surprise; audience: the intelligent

SATIRE: motive/aim: amendment; province: morals & manners; method/means: accentuation; audience: the self-satisfied

SARCASM: motive/aim: inflicting pain; province: faults & foibles; method/means: inversion; audience: victim & bystander

INVECTIVE: motive/aim: discredit; province: misconduct; method/means: direct statement; audience: the public

IRONY: motive/aim: exclusiveness; province: statement of facts; method/means: mystification; audience: an inner circle

CYNICISM: motive/aim: self-justification; province: morals; method/means: exposure of nakedness; audience: the respectable

SARDONIC: motive/aim: self-relief; province: adversity; method/means: pessimism; audience: the self

also from mid-14c.

We alway have to remember the Greeks were educated by the Egyptians, ie…

Eu - Good, Perfect, Complete

Melanin (Melanos) - Black

EuMelanin is the new way to reference Osiris.

The new usage of humor came from state of mind, which came from your health, based in the balance of fluids.

#StayWet

The herbs and bitters are to condition the internal fluids, the BleuMagick conditions the body's waters, we are now going to top it off with #SkinFood, to make sure you can #StayWet.

Please read &/or reread Lymphatic Immunity, Mitochondria Water, HydroChemistry…

You've got to learn everything you can from these books about Water. Then you will be ready to apply these principles and practices, Kitchen Chemistry, Orthorexia & this book espouse! Truth be told, these 3 books are plug and play immediately… but the further study is what refines you. You have to disappear sometime and come back stronger. You don't that by consuming new information in your absence.

The biggest difference between those in the Rat Race, and those who aren't, is Priority of Consuming New Information. Reading.

What does it mean to you that, the other pigments in the skin control Melanin production?

What does it mean to you that, they just discovered 3000 new types of Neurons?

Neurons are either specialized Melanocytes or Melanocytes are specialized Neurons, they have discovered 3,000 new types Naga.... Wake Up!!! Either your whole body is a Brain or a Heart! The Heart has all of these cells, Neurons, Nerves, Melanocytes etc...

What does it mean to you that, they just discovered 135 genes that are associated with Pigment? Is that 135 genes for the Skin? Brain? Heart???

My goal is to make #SkinFood inexpensive enough for you and your family to use twice a day, that way we can #StayWet.

In L'Goat we explain in detail how water builds what it needs, with the right conditions. First thing is well, Water. Second thing obviously is Retinoids, to fertilize the soil. Then of course Sunlight...

You are the Dust of the Ground, Divine Soil, remember that the ground exerts pressure on seeds. You need the proper exercise, to create that mechanical pressure to stimulate growth and regeneration. Mechanical Pressure helps to circulate Magnetism, this is the #BleuMagick of #ElectroMagneticTissue.

If this is your first book of ours that you have read... God Bless Eu, or maybe this isn't your first book but you haven't read PiezoElectroChemistry, please do that...

You are the Fruit of Melanin, your S.elf O.rganizing U.niversal L.ight.

Soul is the Fruit of PhotoVoltaic Pigment.

The Bible has many allusions to the **Sun** and its 12 houses, but they replace the Sun with the Son. The Bible is full of Truth, full of Science, you just have to know what your looking at. Kemetic Science is a mixture of Photochemistry, Photobiology & Acoustics. The key is remembering that Light and Sound only exist in your mind. The electromagnetic spectrum you are used to seeing is deceptive, so I have taken the liberty to provide you with a more straight forward version in this book.

ElectronVolts - an electronvolt (symbol eV, also written electron-volt and electron volt) is the measure of an amount of_**kinetic energy** gained by a single electron accelerating from rest through an electric potential difference of one volt in vacuum, 1 eV equal to the exact value 1.602176634×10−19 J, a unit of energy or work, **the work** required to move an electron through a potential difference of one volt. 1 eV would correspond to an infrared photon of wavelength 1240 nm or frequency 241.8 THz.

4-12 ELECTRON VOLTS = UVC 100-320 NM DEATH WM

3.9 ELECTRON VOLTS = UVB SKIN 290-320 NM

DISEASE JW

3.4 ELECTRON VOLTS = UVA 320-400 NM EYE DISEASE SW

.001 ELECTRON VOLTS = FAR INFRARED 1000000 NM BEYOND THIS POINT IS RADIO WAVES

.4 ELECTRON VOLTS = NEAR FAR INFRARED 3000 NM

.8 ELECTRON VOLTS = MEDIUM INFRARED 1500 NM

1.5 ELECTRON VOLTS = NEAR INFRARED 780 NM

1.7 ELECTRON VOLTS = VISIBLE RED 620-780 NM

2 ELECTRON VOLTS = VISIBLE ORANGE 585-620 NM

2.1 ELECTRON VOLTS = VISIBLE YELLOW 570-585 NM

2.3 ELECTRON VOLTS = VISIBLE GREEN 490-570 NM

2.6 ELECTRON VOLTS = VISIBLE BLUE 440-490 NM

2.9 ELECTRON VOLTS = VISIBLE INDIGO 420-440 NM

3 ELECTRON VOLTS = VISIBLE VIOLET 400-420 NM

We will look at the E.M. Spectrum in terms of Electron Volts, this makes more sense because all of chemistry is based on the movement of electrons. The Sun is the great visible agent of the first cause. This of course means you have to rethink the whole entire ElectroChemistry aka Dr. Sebi vs Dr. EnQi book…

Sound Range: 20 to 20,000 Hz

Voice Range 90 to 255 Hz

Radio Range: 1 hertz up to 3,000 billion hertz. Below Radio is Cellular, Extremely low frequency (ELF) electric and magnetic fields (EMF) occupy the lower part of the electromagnetic spectrum in the frequency range 0-100 kHz. ELF EMF result from electrically charged particles.

Infrared Range 1 Trillion Hertz to … this is where our body heat is…

TECHNOLOGY EQUIPMENT RECAP

HydroGenes - 1! Proton and 1! Electron.

Melanocytes - Photovoltaic Cells

Neurons/Nerves - Electromagnetic Cells

Fascia - Plasma Medium (misonomered Ether)

Brain - CPU, Inductor

Brainstem - Two-way Adapter for CPU into the Motherboard

Pineal Gland - Receiver, Crystal Tuner & Actuator Arm/Head responsible for Phosphorescence, Thermoluminescence, Piezoelectricity, Birefringence & Harmonic Generation (very much like the otoconia in the ears)

Operating System - Deductive Logic or PQ

<u>Heart</u> - Hydraulic Ram, Turbine (from the Greek τύρβη, tyrbē, or Latin turbo, meaning vortex) and Hard Drive.

<u>Melanosomes</u> - Alternators

<u>Mitochondria</u> - Motors

<u>Myelin Sheath</u> - Insulation

<u>Cytoskeleton</u> - Filaments

<u>Phospholipids</u> - Capacitors, Dielectric Material (lipids in general)

<u>Spine</u> - Piezoelectric, Motherboard, Radio Wave Antenna

<u>RBC</u> - Floppy Discs

<u>Lymph Nodes</u> - Filters, Nodes

<u>Tastebuds</u> - Electronic Scanners

<u>Protein</u> - Transformer

<u>Transformers 'Roll Out'</u> - Conformational Change (Macromolecule Shape Shifting)

<u>Antioxidants</u> - Semi-conductors (especially the selenium based...)

<u>Body Cells</u> - Plasma based Crystal disc, fitted with integrated circuits as well as gates and channels (see Human Cell Membrane and/or Computer Chip)

<u>Nerves & Vessels</u> - 'Copper' wires (CoAxial Cables) and Fiber Optics

<u>Pigment, Nerve & Blood Clusters</u> - Input Devices like a Mouse, Keyboard, etc…

<u>DNA</u> - Piezoelectric, Antenna, Data Storing Inductors.

DNA sub entry **<u>Tissues</u>** - Short Living Stories.

DNA sub entry **<u>Genome</u>** - Substrate & Product, a digital Library (HardDrive) of all your Ancestors have ever seen, said, touched, tasted or heard.

DNA sub entry **<u>Chromosome</u>** - Rewritable Unlimited Storage Books (Folders) of the Library, DNA.

DNA sub entry **<u>Histone</u>** - Writing instrument, encoders and **book spines**.

DNA sub entry **<u>non-coding RNA</u>** - Self Organizing Books Shelves

DNA sub entry **<u>Gene</u>** - Chapters (Files) in the Books, source codes.

DNA sub entry **<u>Messenger RNA</u>** - Protein Information, a Sentence.

DNA sub entry **<u>Codon</u>** - Word (Binary Code there are 2 bonds between each 3 nucleotides representing their arrangement), Amino Acid.

DNA sub entry **Nucleotide** - Letter

DNA sub entry **Nucleoside** - Bits of Information

Collagen Based Tissue - Piezoelectric Inductors

Stomach - Chemical Mixer

Lumen - the SI unit of luminous flux = to the amount of light emitted per second..... or hollow structures in vessels and cells... hmmm????

Eyes - Camera Lens/Charge Coupled Device (CCD), Digital to Analogue Converter, Complex Photovoltaic Cells/Photodetector...

Amino Acids - Fuses that can be almost anything!

Nucleic Acid - Actual Intelligence (self powering too).

N-Type Semiconductors - Selenium or Silica doped with Phosphorus (Alkaline-ish)

P-Type Semiconductors - Selenium or Silica doped with Boron (Acid-ish)

PN Junction - <u>Crystal Lattice Structure</u> Material allowing the flowing of electrons in one direction.

Bone and Fascia seem to be a massive N-Type, P-Type, PN Junction Super computer on it's own... especially if we add in the Piezoelectricity & Vitamin D!

<u>Rectifier</u> - N-Type + P-Type + PN Junction in Bone

<u>Melanin</u> - CPU Core, Solar Repeater

<u>Human Cell Membrane and/or Computer Chip</u> - A flat semiconducting (crystal) disc or wafer, with integrated circuits (resistors/conductors) and/or gates & channels. We now have to add the filaments into this Crystal Disc we call a Body Cell or Somatic Cell.

<u>Transistors</u> - a semiconductor device with three connections, capable of amplification in addition to rectification.

The location that a virus goes viral in, is called a **<u>Hotspot</u>**? WTH!

<u>Virus</u> - an infective agent that typically consists of a nucleic acid molecule in a protein coat, is too small to be seen by light microscopy, and is able to multiply only within the living cells of a host.

Wait you see that, it is happening again! Host...

See look there is another definition of **<u>Virus</u>** - a piece of code that is capable of copying itself and typically has a detrimental effect, such as corrupting the system or destroying data.

Wait a damn minute! DNA is a piece of **<u>code</u>**... A viral strand of DNA or RNA that can jump host is fully capable in that context of copying itself, one would even argue, that is it's only 'motion'. The detrimental effects of corrupting the system (physical illness) or destroying data (mental illness), can clearly be seen anthropomorphically.

Alien - Virus

Culture - the arts and other manifestations of human intellectual achievement regarded collectively, the customs, arts, social institutions, and achievements of a particular nation, people, or other social group. The cultivation of bacteria, tissue cells, etc. in an artificial medium containing nutrients, a preparation of cells obtained from a culture. The cultivation of **plants**.

Going Live - become operational.

Live Stream - a live transmission of an event over the internet, transmit or receive live video and audio coverage of (an event) over the internet.

The Web - Arachnoid Mater

Download - copy (data) from one computer system to another, typically over the internet, an act or process of downloading data.

Upload - transfer (data) from one computer to another, typically to one that is larger or remote from the user or functioning as a server, an act or process of downloading data.

Data - facts and statistics collected together for reference or analysis; the quantities, characters, or symbols on which operations are performed by a computer, being stored and transmitted in the form of electrical signals and recorded on magnetic, optical, or mechanical recording media.

Host - an animal or plant on or in which a parasite or commensal organism lives. VS

Host - store (a website or other data) on a server or other computer so that it can be accessed over the internet.

Transmission is the act of transferring something from one spot to another, like a radio or TV broadcast, or a disease going from one person to another.

I am highlighting the unknown and proposing we may have some answers! Infection - an infectious disease.

plural noun: infections "a chest infection"

Vs

Infection - the presence of a virus in, or its introduction into, a computer system. What is a computer system?

Computer System - a computer system is a programmable electronic device that can accept input; store data; and retrieve, process and output information.

<u>Pandemic language = Virology/Biology language.</u> The question is, why? The next question is what does that have to do with Dr. Sebi or Robert Becker? The obvious....

<u>Computer System</u> - a computer system is a programmable electronic device that can accept input; store data; and retrieve, process and output information.

<u>Computer System</u> - a single information processor but usually a group of processors that have specified and general computations; grouped by hardware ie... liver cells, lung cells, brain cells etc.. What you think?

<u>Exercise</u> - activity requiring physical effort, carried out to sustain or improve health and fitness. "exercise improves your heart and lung power"

<u>Exercise</u> - computer training or computer based training.

<u>Exigenetics</u> - Term created by Dr. EnQi for Melanin vs Diabetes research, denoting the control that exercise has over gene expression.

<u>Hydration</u> - the process of inducing gelling, ionizing, dissolution & turbulent flow with activation of cytochrome c (via infrared light).

<u>Resonance</u> - the quality in a sound of being deep, full, and reverberating. "the resonance of his voice"

- The ability to evoke or suggest images, memories, and emotions."the concepts lose their emotional resonance"

- The reinforcement or prolongation of sound by reflection from a surface or by the synchronous vibration of a neighboring object.

- The condition in which an electric circuit or device produces the largest possible response to an applied oscillating signal, especially when its inductive and its capacitative reactances are balanced.

- The condition in which an object or system is subjected to an oscillating force having a frequency close to its own natural frequency.

- The occurrence of a simple ratio between the periods of revolution of two bodies about a single primary.

- The state attributed to certain molecules of having a structure that cannot adequately be represented by a single structural formula but is a composite of two or more structures of higher energy.

- • A short-lived subatomic particle that is an excited state of a more stable particle.

Induction - the action or process of inducting someone to a position or organization."the league's induction into the Baseball Hall of Fame"

Induction - a formal introduction to a new job or position.plural noun: inductions
"an induction course"
enlistment into military service.

Induction - The process or action of bringing about or giving rise to something."isolation, starvation, and other forms of stress induction" the process of bringing on childbirth or abortion by artificial means, typically by the use of drugs.

Induction - The inference of a general law from particular instances.

Induction -"the admission that laws of nature cannot be established by induction" the production of facts to prove a general statement.

Induction - a means of proving a theorem by showing that if it is true of any particular case it is true of the next case in a series, and then showing that it is indeed true in one particular case.

Induction - noun: mathematical induction; plural noun: mathematicals inductionthe production of an electric or magnetic state by the proximity (without contact) of an electrified or magnetized body.

Induction - The production of an electric current in a conductor by varying the magnetic field applied to the conductor.

Induction - The stage of the working cycle of an internal combustion engine in which the fuel mixture is drawn into the cylinders.

Is there anyone reading this that would disagree with our body fitting these definitions, the definitions of a computer?

Man this thought experiment just got a lot more interesting didn't it? MIT and the US Military are different types of receipts huh? Is it possible frequency resonance, spreads disease? Human modems? Can Shedding be a broadcast signal?

Wi-Fi is a wireless networking technology that uses radio waves to provide wireless high-speed Internet access. A common misconception is that the term **Wi-Fi** is short for "wireless fidelity," however Wi-Fi is a trademarked phrase that refers to IEEE 802.11x standards.

Viral shedding is a term for when viruses are replicating or reproducing, the virus is being led out of the host cell where it's replicating or

reproducing ... Viral shedding is the expulsion and release of virus progeny following successful reproduction during a host cell infection. Once replication has been completed and the host cell is exhausted of all resources in making viral progeny, the viruses may begin to leave the cell by several methods.

Vaccine - a substance used to stimulate immunity to a particular infectious disease or pathogen, typically prepared from
an inactivated or weakened form of the causative agent or from
its constituents or products.

Vaccine - a program designed to detect computer viruses and inactivate them.

"the rate of use of vaccines for computer viruses is not as high as in the US, Japan, and other countries"

Application - a medicinal substance put on the skin.

Application - a program or piece of software designed and written to fulfill a particular purpose of the user.

In our thought experiment, if a virus is simply the

media for harmful information...

<u>Media</u> - an intermediate layer in the wall of a blood vessel or lymphatic vessel.

<u>Media</u> - the main means of mass communication (broadcasting, publishing, and the internet) regarded collectively.

<u>DOPE</u> - an illicit drug (such as heroin or cocaine) used for its intoxicating or euphoric effects
especially : MARIJUANA (dopamine altering)

<u>Dope</u> - a preparation (such as an anabolic steroid, diuretic, or tranquilizer) given to a racehorse to help or hinder its performance

<u>To Dope</u> - In semiconductor production, to dope is the intentional introduction of impurities into an intrinsic semiconductor for the purpose of modulating its electrical, optical and structural properties. The doped material is referred to as an extrinsic semiconductor.

<u>Short Circuit</u> - Cardiac Arrest?

<u>Short Circuit</u> - Multiple Sclerosis (due to loss of insulation)

<u>Overheating</u> - Fever?

<u>Overcurrent</u> - Inflammation

With Infection and Virus included we are onto

something.

<u>Current</u> - belonging to the present time; happening or being used or done now.

<u>Current</u> - <u>a body of water</u> or air <u>moving in</u> <u>a</u> *definite* <u>direction</u>, especially <u>through a surrounding body of water</u> or air in which there is less movement.

<u>Current</u> - a flow of electricity that results from the ordered directional movement of electrically charged particles.

<u>Current</u> - a quantity representing the rate of flow of electric charge, usually measured in amperes.

<u>Current</u> - the general tendency or course of events or opinion.

<u>Leakage Current</u> - the unintended loss of energy, gain of resistance or results of faulty/worn out insulation.

<u>Plasma</u> - Electric Currents or Electric Current Carrier

<u>Electric Current</u> - Magnetic Field (AtomSphere) Carrier

<u>Alternating Magnetic & Electric Waves</u> - Light

<u>NeuroTransmitters</u> - Record of ElectroMagnetic Waves produced by Neurons (ElectroChemical Message)

<u>Hormones</u> - Large simple versions of NeuroTransmitters (ElectroChemical Message)

<u>Malware</u> - External Negative Mental Programming

<u>Food</u> - Informative Electronic Batteries

0) Movement and sound create energy from water for basic cellular function, via the EnQi Cycle which includes Mitochondria Water. This system slowly increases as all other energy systems fail.

1) Phosphocreatine - anaerobic (no respiration required), phosphocreatine donates it "phospho" to ADP to recycle ATP. This makes 10 ATP per second, its a 1 to 1 ratio (1 phosphocreatine creates 1 ATP) and this is the jump start energy.

2) Anaerobic Glycolysis - anaerobic (no respiration required), Glycogen &/or Glucose to Lactate, 5 ATP per second, 1 to 3 ratio (1 Glycogen creates 3 ATP while 1 Glucose creates 2 ATP) and this is bulk of the energy we focus on, 9 - 120 seconds.

3) NAD/Cytochrome 1 - aerobic (requires oxygen), Glycogen &/or Glucose to CO_2/H_2O, 2.5 ATP per second, 1 to 38 ratio (1 Glycogen &/or Glucose creates 38 ATP), 2 minutes up to 2 hours.

4) FAD/Cytochrome 2 - aerobic (requires oxygen), FFA &/or Triglycerides to CO_2/H_2O, 1.5 ATP per second, 1 to 360 ratio (1 Glycogen &/or Glucose creates 360 ATP), 2 minutes up to 2 days.

Food rule of thumb - Resynthesis of ATP of Inverse to Yield, the closer the ratio is to 1:1 the fast it can be recycled.

Muscle rule of thumb - Frequently used muscle is slow twitch, Fast twitch is slowly used (at that's the blueprint).

Electric Power - the **rate** at which work is done or energy is transformed into an electrical circuit. Simply put, it is a measure of how much energy is used in a span of time.

Conductor - a person who directs the performance of an orchestra or choir.

Conductor - a material or device that conducts or transmits heat, electricity, or sound, especially when regarded in terms of its capacity to do this.

Lymphatic System - Watermill

Circulatory System - Generator

Integumentary System - Photovoltaic Diaphragm

Immune System - Antivirus, Malware Scanner, Frequency Filter & Rectifier

Nervous System - Power Transmission and Cellular Communications Lines

<u>Fascia System</u> - HydroElectric Grid, Scaffolding

<u>Respiratory System</u> - Windmill

<u>Windmill</u> - a structure that converts wind power or "air" power into rotational energy or vortex energy, to mill grain. In our case grain is Magnetism!

MAGNETS ARE DEFINED BY GRAINS
MAGNETIC GRAINS ARE DEFINED BY APPLIED
STRESS AND CRYSTAL GEOMETRY
SPM SUPERMAGNETIC
SD SINGLE DOMAIN
PSD PSEUDO DOMAIN
MD MULTIDOMAIN

<u>Reproductive System</u> - Quine (self-replicating programs)

<u>Skeletal System</u> - Piezoelectric Crystal Shaped to produced highly specific frequency under stress, Dynamic Oscillators.

<u>Urinary System</u> - Industrial Wastewater, Return Flow, Surface Runoff, Urban Runoff Agricultural & Animal Husbandry Wastewater

<u>Digestive System</u> - Massive Inductor

<u>Mouth</u> - Industrial Grinder

<u>Endocrine System</u> - Programmer for Human Cell Membrane and/or Crystal Gel Computer Chips

<u>Human Being</u> - Resonator

<u>Vessels</u> - Pipes

<u>Aromatic Ring</u> - Cyclotron (Particle Accelerator)

<u>Glycation</u> - Corrosion

<u>Exegenetics</u> - Holistic Biomechanics; the purposeful science of combining light, water, diet & exercise to effect DNA.

<u>EnQi's 1st Law of Metabolism</u> - The conversion rate of cholesterol should match the activity of Melanin in the skin. These two systems are designed to be and stay coupled. A dark skin person with low sunlight intake and low exercise is going to die from a Metabolic Complication. The only time Animal Flesh is safe to be consumed by a Eumelanin Dominant person is in times of starvation or extremely high activity.

This Law is a Constant and when broken results in disease every time.

<u>EnQi's 2nD Law of Metabolism</u> - The average rate of applied mechanical stress on the bone electrically stimulating bone marrow, determines the rate of bone deterioration and Red Blood Cell production.

<u>EnQi's 3rd Law of Metabolism</u> - The human body metabolizes Transverse Waves and Mechanical Waves into Electricity. Electricity is the main driver of Biochemistry. Exercise is just as potent a driver of Biochemistry as the Sun.

<u>EnQi's 4th Law of Metabolism</u> - Electron movement and bonding is the Nature of Chemistry. PhotoChemistry and PiezoElectroChemistry are the Primary drivers of Biochemistry.

The Ancients discovered this and created Martial Artforms as a way to clean the Bone, Bone Marrow & Brain. Plaque & Sugar are the top drivers of Brain Disease. The things destroying the Heart are secondarily destroying the brain, and they are the breaking of these Universal Laws.

<u>EnQi's 5th Law of Metabolism</u> - Nutrients are actually substrates that must be transformed via biochemistry to be meaningful. This means that providing your body with lots of nutrition without the Water, Light & Exercise don't work alone.

<u>EnQi's 6th Law of Metabolism</u> - The Body maintains the least amount of bone marrow required to handle blood demand. The marrow is very energy demanding, thus attracting and storing fat for energy, eventually becoming fat itself. Fatty bone marrow is called yellow bone marrow. Yellow Bone Marrow can be reconverted to Red Bone Marrow should the body's demands require it, and the body's resources facilitate it. The primary driver is pressure, hormesis training on the Bones. BMR is heavily driven by Bone Marrow, this means Bone Marrow is a driver if insulin and insulin resistance.

<u>EnQi's 7th Law of Metabolism</u> - The system of pigments throughout the body are for metabolism of Light, actual Soulfood. The Adsorption & Absorption of Photons by Water.

Adsorption - increase in the concentration of a dissolved substance at the interface of a condensed and a liquid phase due to the operation of surface forces.

Absorption - a physical or chemical phenomenon or a process in which atoms, molecules or ions enter some bulk phase – liquid or solid material. This is a different process from adsorption, since molecules undergoing absorption are taken up by the volume, not by the surface.

<u>EnQi's 8th Law of Metabolism</u> - in a diabetic state, sugar is simply invisible to the body. Sugar is not being "sensed" because it's not being converted to energy. In this state of starvation the body turns on every pathway it has to produce sugar from everything you have in your body, fats and proteins included.

This is the reason that it seems like no matter what you eat or 'don't eat', your blood sugar goes up. It's very frustrating. The only way to make it stop is converting that substrate (glucose) into it's final product (energy). The reception of the actual energy, tells the body to stop producing substrate, we good. This must start in the legs and back, the largest muscles but most overlooked. The legs are particularly punished by sitting for extended periods of time, 3-6 hours straight, for a total over 3/4 the time your awake! The leg circulation atrophies and destroys the nerves, nerves are neurons that need a lot of nutrients!

*You must cross reference any and all protocols; food, exercise, medication etc... with the Constitution book & Declaration of Independence!

EnQi Prayer
Hail SHU who Created the Heavens & the Earth, Hail Wusir who gave us Pigment.
And there was Electromagnetic Waves, before and beyond our pigment created Light, for which we give thanks.
And there was Mechanical Waves, before and beyond our pigment created Sound, for which we give thanks.
And there is heat, for which we are grateful.
And there is power, for which we are grateful.
Blessed be Tefnuit & Nuit, for giving us a womb made of water.
Blessed be Shu & Geb, who gave us ElectroMagnetism.
Blessed be Djehuti, who gave us wisdom.
Blessed be Atum-Re, who gave us sight.
We give thanks for the Blessings of Shu.

Blessed are we for cellular E.L.F waves, so our cells can talk to each other.

Blessed are we for long radio waves, which oscillate slowly.

Blessed are we for broadcast waves, for which we educate & communicate with via Djed Pillars natural and handmade.

Blessed are we for short waves, linkers of humankind.

Blessed are we for microwaves, that we may sea better.

Blessed are we for infrared, bearers of nourishing heat and Melatonin.

Blessed are we for visible light, tuned to our waters.

Blessed are we for red, sacred to Set.

Blessed are we for orange (dark yellow there was no orange in Kemet), sacred to the Rising Sun.

Blessed are we for Khenet (yellow), hallowed by Re's gaze.

Blessed are we for sWadj (green), the color of our skin, gift from Wusir.

Blessed are we for Khesbedj (lazuli Blue), for its hydrogen line and recycling Vitamin A.

Blessed are we for Irtyu (indigo), which tricks us by looking mefkhat (turquoise) sometime.

Blessed are we for violet, flourishing with energy.

Blessed are we for ultraviolet, which creates Melanin & Vitamin D.

Blessed are we for X rays, sacred to stone, that we

may sea better.

Blessed are we for the gamma, dangerously high vibrations.

We give thanks for the Geniuses Tesla, Mesmer, Swan, Brush, Planck, Einstein, Thomas, Heaviside, Steinmetz, West, Brown (a sister), Easley (a sister), Morgan (Black Edison), Latimer, Sampson, Russell, Turner, Sebi, Becker and others that re-membered the body of Shu-Amun for us.

In light of Light and Sound, in light of Electromagnetic Waves, Mechanical Waves and the Holy Trinity, Amen!

BOOKS

ELECTRICIAN'S RADIO ANATOMY MANUAL
GOAT VS BAPHOMET
THEY NOT LIKE US
Chase DuQuesnay Dr. EnQi ReaL

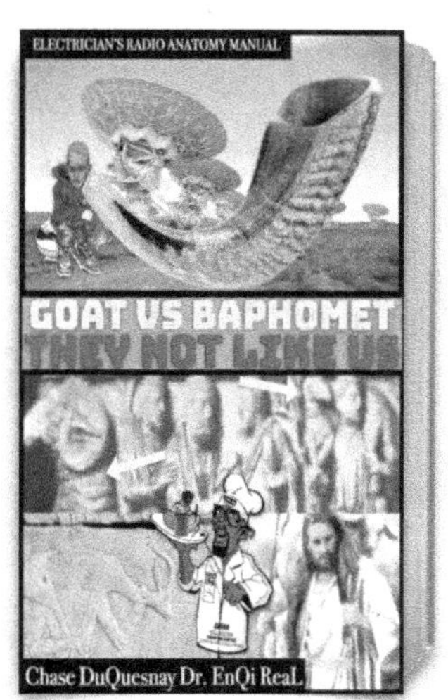

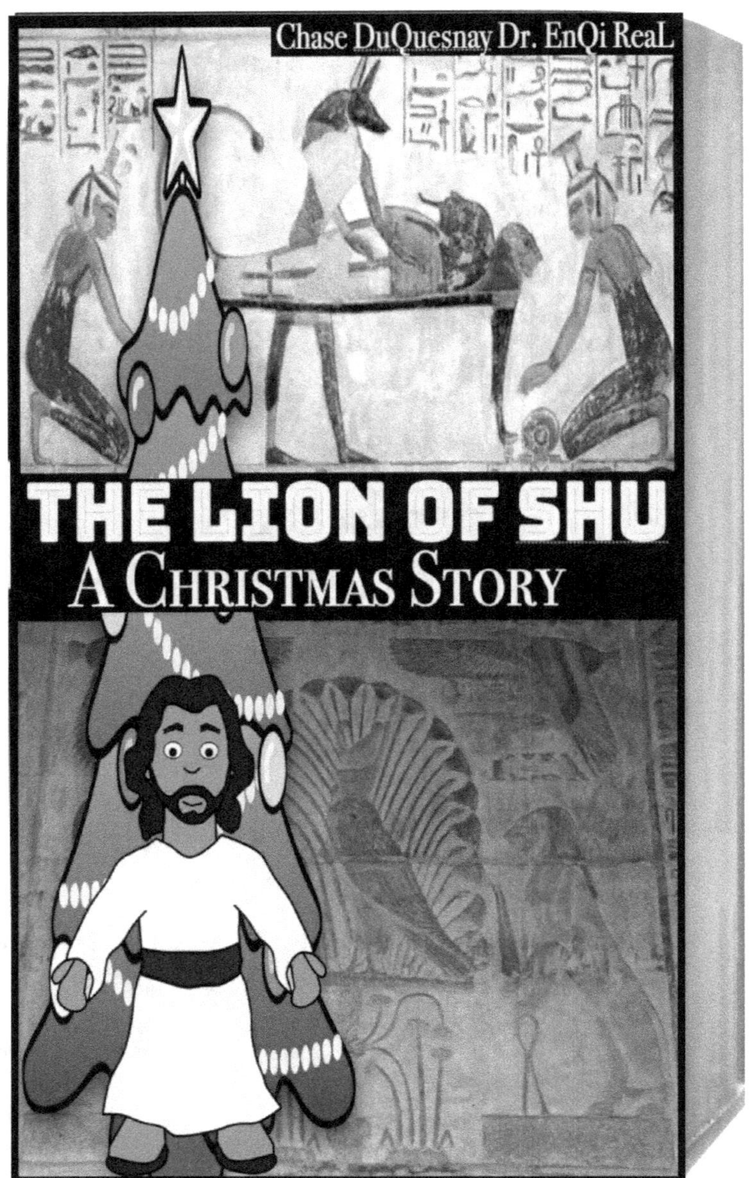

Chase DuQuesnay Dr. EnQi ReaL
THE LION OF SHU
A CHRISTMAS STORY

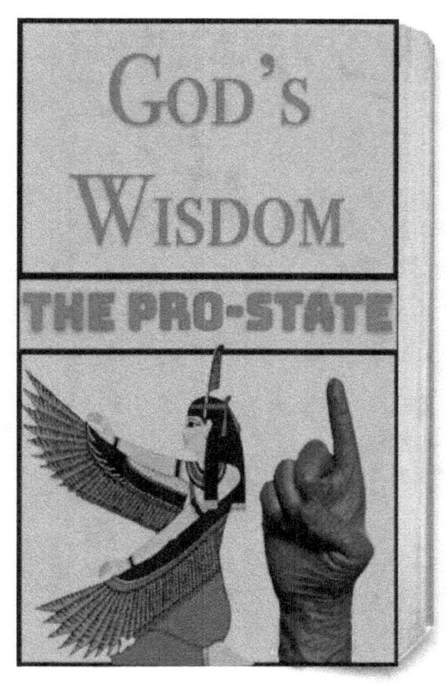

GOD'S
WISDOM
THE PRO-STATE

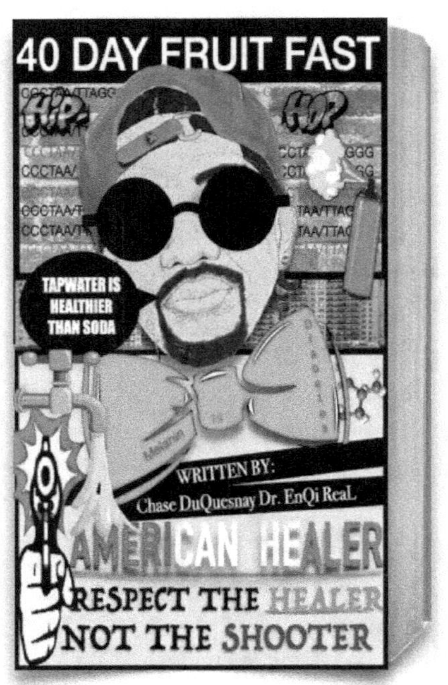

40 DAY FRUIT FAST
HIP
HOP
TAPWATER IS HEALTHIER THAN SODA
WRITTEN BY:
Chase DuQuesnay Dr. EnQi ReaL
AMERICAN HEALER
RESPECT THE HEALER
NOT THE SHOOTER

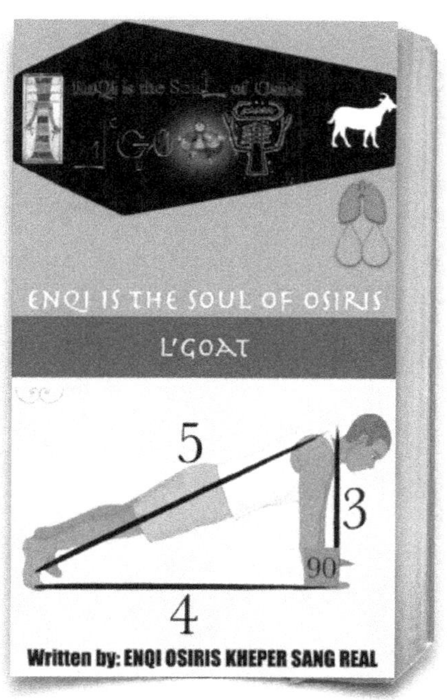
ENQI IS THE SOUL OF OSIRIS
L'GOAT
5
3
90
4
Written by: ENQI OSIRIS KHEPER SANG REAL